# Two Day Diet

## Permanent Plan for Fast Weight Loss

By Peter Kornfeld
Copyright © 2013

# Income Disclaimer

This book contains business strategies, marketing methods and other business advice that, regardless of my own results and experience, may not produce the same results (or any results) for you. I make absolutely no guarantee, expressed or implied, that by following the advice below you will make any money or improve current profits, as there are several factors and variables that come into play regarding any given business.

Primarily, results will depend on the nature of the product or business model, the conditions of the marketplace, the experience of the individual, and situations and elements that are beyond your control.

As with any business endeavor, you assume all risk related to investment and money based on your own discretion and at your own potential expense.

# Liability Disclaimer

By reading this book, you assume all risks associated with using the advice given below, with a full understanding that you, solely, are responsible for anything that may occur as a result of putting this information into action in any way, and regardless of your interpretation of the advice.

You further agree that our company cannot be held responsible in any way for the success or failure of your business as a result of the information presented in this book. It is your responsibility to conduct your own due diligence regarding the safe and successful operation of your business if you intend to apply any of our information in any way to your business operations.

## Terms of Use

You are given a non-transferable, "personal use" license to this book. You cannot distribute it or share it with other individuals.

Also, there are no resale rights or private label rights granted when purchasing this book. In other words, it's for your own personal use only.

# Two Day Diet

## Permanent Plan for Fast Weight Loss

By Peter Kornfeld

# Table of Contents

# Introduction

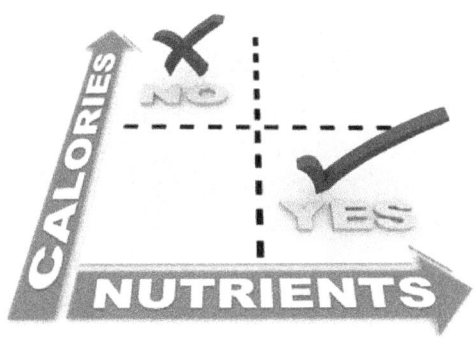

Diets seem to come and go. There's always a new "Fad" diet that claims to zap fat overnight and leave you slimmer, sexier and happier with little or no effort. When push comes to shove pretty much all of it is gibberish. If something seems too good to be true, it's likely not.
But as a lazy society that's greedy in general, we want so badly to believe in these ludicrous diets that we consciously convince ourselves to "give it a shot". Truly believing this is the diet that will make us beautiful forever without any sacrifice or effort.

WAKE UP CALL! FAD DIETS DO NOT WORK NO MATTER WHICH WAY YOU SLICE THEM.

Common sense diets that teach healthy eating and smart exercising are going to get you the results you desire if you are patient, persistent, consistent and you don't quit! Initially this "Two Day Diet" was created as a section of a medical plan to help reduce the risk of breast cancer. It didn't take long for experts to see this diet offered a sensible approach to eating that could help people drop fat, build their body strong, steer off serious disease, and make this a healthy choice for life. Talk about hitting the jackpot!

The "Two Day Diet" works because it's been practiced by Mediterranean's for years, it's proven. It uses common sense nutritional logic, with a firm understanding of how the body works and why it needs specific vitamins and minerals on a regular basis every day, not just when you get around to it.

Finally, there's a diet that actually works and sets you up for long-term success. It's not just a romp in the hay that comes and goes and leaves you with nothing. Not only is this diet or new eating strategy sensible, but it also gives you protective health benefits en route. Something the majority of diets lack because they are stressing and depriving your body of key vital nutrients in the hopes of zapping fat and getting your skinning, regardless of the cost to your overall good health. Now that doesn't make any sense does it?

Well there's no use crying over spilt milk is there. Let's leave the past in the past and move forward with the key to your sustainable weight loss and long-term good health, "The Two Day Diet."

# Two Day Diet Works - Why?

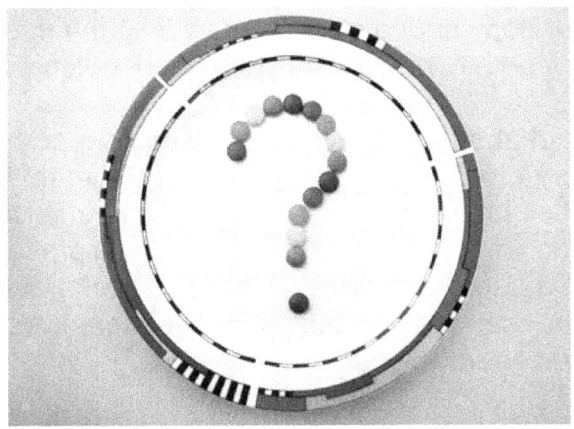

It's created to decrease your natural appetite, leaving you less hungry, while making sure you are getting all the essential vitamins and minerals your body requires, and optimizing fat burn while preserving muscle.

I hate to be the bearer of bad new but you can't physiologically lose weight simply by eating healthy 2 days and pigging out for 5! Don't despair because you still get to eat "freely" for 5 days, but with "healthy" in mind.

If you want to lose weight you need to fuel our body with the essential macronutrients (protein and carbs), vitamins and minerals ALWAYS. It's very important to ensure that even on your "restrictive" healthy days you get all the nutrients your body needs. If you don't you are just opening the door for all sorts of issues to start manifesting; disease, mood swings, low energy, aches/pains, poor sleep, and so forth.

Two Day Diet is logical and scientifically based. It was created to make certain you drop pesky fat but also don't deprive yourself to get the wanted results. In other words I need to make it loud and clear that you can lose fat and build your body strong without neglecting the nutrients your body relies on every day for overall optimal health.

If that's not enough, 40+ years of history supports this diet theory - High Protein and Low Fat Vegetables and Fruit = Weight Loss! This is the way the Mediterranean's have done it for years. Further still, studies prove the Two Day Diet deters heart disease, cancer, stroke, and so many other serious diseases that take more lives need-lessly than I care to count.

The concept is basic healthy eating always with 2 days of "calculated" but healthy restriction in order to reach and maintain your ideal weight. Based on milk, fruits and vegetables - with the milk giving you calcium, protein and numerous other vitamins, helping you to feel full, whilst the fruit and fresh vegetables give you the fiber and other nutrients your body needs to get healthy.

How about we validate this diet with some scientific fact? The Science Behind The 2 Day Diet!
It's fair to wonder "why" this diet is going to work when all others have failed. Why is this diet "the one?"

For one this dieting approach isn't just about the calories. Sure the number of calories you consume as a whole is reflective of your weight, along with what kind of calories they are. The key here is bringing to light the psychology of weight loss. In other words your head has to be on board if you want to succeed in long-term weight-loss and wellness.

By having two days where you are restricted considerably in your eating, most would expect a pig-out session extraordinaire on day three. Well this doesn't happen because the mind is okay with giving a little to get a lot.

Your head knows by day three that you've already survived the "tough" part of the diet and it's smooth sailing to the finish line, or at least for five days before you've got to restrict yourself again. And because you've restricted your body you feel really special and satiated when you are actually able to eat larger amounts of healthy foods. This eliminates the feeling of deprivation that sets most fad diets up for failure. With many, it's a never-ending feeling of "not having,"which is just not the case with the "Two Day Diet."

Would you rather two days of healthy and balanced deprivation or deprivation forever? I think you get the picture here.

This strategy also teaches you to stop and smell the rose and appreciate healthy eating by doing. If you can have more of a healthy food choice most of the time and lose weight, that's what you are going to learn to "want" to do over time. With this diet you are never eating loads of high-fat, high calorie foods that don't fill you up and make you fat. Instead you're eating lower calorie nutritionally dense foods that fill you up, keep you energized, help you lose weight and teach you healthy eating. This helps you to unlearn your poor eating habits and create new ones.

Believe it or not the way you eat was learned by you and only you can change it.
It's a common sense diet? Who would have thought?

*My Thoughts . . .*

*It's mind over matter here with a little bit of logic and sci-ence thrown in. Your goal is to change your thinking on eating and make this transition as painless as possible. Obviously the route you've been taking just isn't leaving you feeling happy, sexy and excited for life. The "Two Day Diet" has the tools to help strengthen your mental and physical. It not only shows you why this diet works but how. Having the knowledge and know-how to make positive health changes, particularly with your eating, is the first step in transforming you into everything you know you can be and more. Just a thought . . .*

# How Your Body Burns Fat

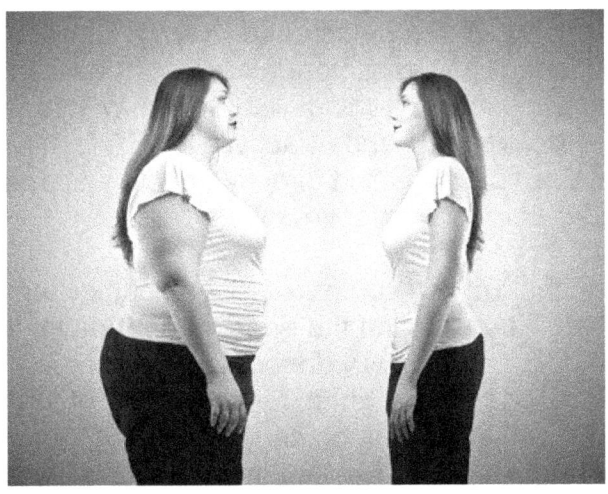

If you are looking to zap fat it's important you understand the basics behind how your body burns it. That just makes sense.

Your body has to burn calories in order to burn fat. This means it needs to burn up or use calories. Calories are simply a measure of energy. It's the same thing as a pound is a measure of weight and a liter is a measure of liquid. If you want to get technical a calorie is measuring how much energy is required to alter the temperature of a gram of water by one degree Celsius. This may not make a whole lot of sense because neither you nor I, are a block of ice. Regardless, this is what a calorie means.

The rate in which you burn up this expendable energy is called metabolism. Defined it's the number of calories your body needs to burn in order to maintain itself. To put this into perspective, you are burning calories continuously whether you are walking, sleeping, eating or exercising.

This is interlinking with fat burning. You are going to have to burn more calories or increase your metabolism in order to lose fat. That said, your metabolic rate is unique to you. It is dependent on things like height, weight, body composition, health, gender, activity level, lifestyle and the exercise you do, which directly affects your metabolism and determines what your weight is.

Your metabolism is a complex process of biochemical processes. Keep in mind the energy your body needs to function in the basic really doesn't alter that much. Your basil metabolic rate accounts for up to 70% of the energy your body burns and can be configured using a formula. We just aren't going to get into that right now. But 2 other factors that influence your metabolism are: thermogenisis and physical activity.

Thermogenisis is the breakdown of food. This includes chewing, swallowing, digestion, absorption and transportation of the fuel to the awaiting organs and internal bodily systems for use. Experts agree that about ten percent of the calories you burn each day are used in thermogenisis.

Exercise is the physical activity you do in order to help your body function optimally. Simple examples are playing basketball, running, biking, playing tag with the kids or swimming. Physical activity is the most changing or variable factor when configuring your metabolism. The more you exercise the more fat and calories you burn and the higher your metabolism. If you sit on your butt, then you aren't burning any calories or increasing your metabolism, making it very difficult for your body to burn excess fat and calories.

Can You Blame Weight Gain on Slow Metabolism?
Sorry, for the most part this excuse is a copout. Your metabolism is a natural process and usually the body is programmed to ensure it balances with the needs of your body. One reason why if you try and restrict your caloric intake with fad diets, not giving your body enough energy to function, your metabolism will intrinsically slow down to try and burn less calories. This is a survival technique you don't want to happen, but your body doesn't trust you and is trying to burn as little energy as possible so you survive. You need to eat in order to lose weight.

Specialty Note: There are medical conditions that are rare that slow your metabolism and cause weight gain, two of which are hypothyroidism and Cushing's syndrome. So why do we gain weight? Well we eat more energy than we burn.

BURNING FAT
Now you really don't have a whole lot of control over your metabolism. But you do have the wheel when it comes to how many calories you burn overall each day. Your physical activity level comes into play here.

You can burn more calories and if you are also eating healthy and consuming the "right" number of food calories each day, the following exercise is going to encourage your body to burn fat.

*| Weight Lifting or Strength Training
* Cardiovascular Activity on a Routine Basis
* Adjustments in Your Everyday - things like taking the stairs and biking to work

We're going to rewind a little bit here back to your digestive metabolism or the energy you utilize to digest and process food. The act of transforming complex carbs into sugar and protein into amino acids for energy, taking up about 10-15% of the total energy you use each day. Interestingly, burning protein uses up more energy than breaking down and transporting carbohydrates does. To bring this to light, burning protein takes about 25 out of every 100 calories. The breaking down of carbohydrates uses up approximately 10 calories out of every 100 calories. It makes sense theoretically to make your body burn more energy with protein right?

Fat burning enzymes in your body are lost very fast. Just think "getting out of shape" here. This causes your muscles to temporarily lose their drive to burn fat, the primary source of fuel for your body. It makes sense that larger people burn more calories than smaller people because there is more effort required in everything.

When it comes to burning fat through exercise, the harder and longer you go the less fat calories you're burning. Instead your energy is coming from mainly sugar, suggesting that shorter exercise with diversity, bursts of energy sporadically seems to be most efficient in triggering your system to burn fat. Great examples are interval training with bouts of cardiovascular activity, alternated with strength training exercises and weights.

The bottom line is that your metabolism, the rate in which your body burns calories, decides if your body is going to burn fat, lose weight, how much and at what speed.

*My Thoughts . . .*
*Knowing how to technically burn fat is only going to give you more power in blasting that pesky fat. If you know how to run to know you can get to the finish line. It's the*

18

*same sort of thinking here. By understanding your metabolism and how it works you can use this information to get to it!*

# Two Restricted Days Explained

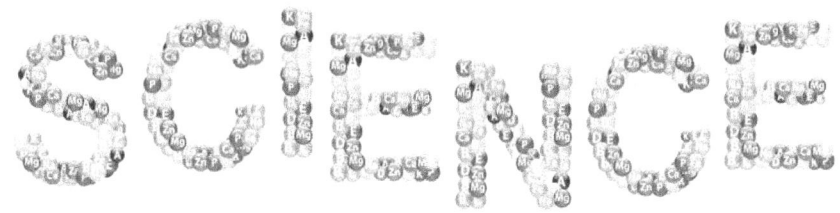

The idea here is to give your body the nutrients it requires while optimizing fat burning.

First we're going to have a look at diversity because this is your friend when it comes to getting healthy, losing weight, toning up and getting results.

You've likely heard about people that have been on diets or exercise programs to lose fat and they're frustratingly hit a plateau. This just means they are putting in the effort, doing all the right things to lose weight and their either slowed or stopped seeing progress. Problem with that is this is what often sends people over the edge and they quit. And who could blame them?

If you're working your butt off exercising religiously 5 days a week and making most of the "right" food choices but not seeing the fat melt off AND you're feeling de-energized and lousy because of this, it's pretty tough to stay mentally sound and stick with the program.
Well if you practice the art of diversity in everything you do, chances are pretty good you are always going to get results. The "Two Day Diet" is a perfect example of this.

In eating you are always changing things up so that your body and mind are always guessing as to what you are going to feed it. This means your body isn't going to get bored and lazy in burning fat and calories. Alternating between having more and less food to burn, and a variety of foods is going to encourage your metabolism to get stuck in high gear. If your metabolism is working harder for you all the time, you are going to burn fat more effectively and efficiently.

Diversity is the key in helping you reach your fat-loss goals and so much more - believe it!

Now that we understand the importance of diversity, let's move more into what the 2 days of restrictive eating is all about.

The 2 days of restrictive eating are necessary because you do need to curb your eating if you want to lose weight. What happens is many find it really hard to "diet" for 7 days. So the "Two Day Diet" sets you up for success by helping you lose weight and only have 2 days where you really need to watch what you eat. It's a definite bargain for perpetual dieters.

Your mind is a powerful thing and by making your head happy, your body often follows. There's no need to worry about depriving your body of nutrients on these days because this diet was created by dieticians. So it's nutritionally sound and many find it really easy to stick to just because it's simple.

On these two days you eat significantly less calories but still give your body the basics of what it needs to function. On these two days you eat around 650 calories, depending on your height, weight, age,exercise level and body composition. A nutritionist can help you detail this or you can plug it into a formula online and get a pretty good idea of what you need. These two days of restriction gives your mind the ability to accept you are dieting, but in moderation. Meaning you are eating a little bit less than you might like to but only for two days, which is reasonable in the scheme of a week.

On these two days you are only allowed to eat . . .
* 2 cups of low-fat milk or the same in cottage cheese or yogurt
* A minimum of 2 cups low-calorie drinks, including tea, coffee, flavored water, water, sugar-free carbonated drinks
* 1 serving fruit
* 4 servings vegetables or salad
* Multi-vitamin
So what do you do if you don't like milk?
You can substitute each third of a cup for . . .
* 100 g cottage cheese
* 100g yogurt
* 150g low-fat yogurt

Yes the ingredients on these 2 restrictive days aren't ample, but you can make things a little more exciting with a little imagination. Things work like . . .
* Creamy veggie soup
* Spice up your milk with cinnamon. or nutmeg
* Fruit smoothies are great
* Fruit added to yogurt or cottage cheese

Food Further
Most fruits and vegetables you can have, except high-calorie fruit juices that are loaded with sugars. You should also avoid the following foods just on the two days because they are very high in calories:
- parsnips and potatoes

- avocado and sweet potato
- beans and pulses
- dried fruit and plantain
- yams

For flavoring you are safe to go with:
- garlic, chili and spices
- herbs, lime and lemon juice
- Worcester sauce, vinegar

*My Thinking . . .*
*Losing weight and getting healthy is a give and take relationship, same as everything else. You can opt to succeed and understand you need to work a little harder with your eating two out of seven days. Or you can set yourself up to fail with another fad diet that seems too good to be true. Think of it like giving two dollars to get five. Pretty good deal if you ask me.*

*Sure you may not be eating as much as you'd like on these two days, but it's necessary if you are going to re-program your brain to appreciate eating healthy food in moderation. For bonus even though you are eating quite a bit less than you might normally, you're still giving your body all the nutrition it requires and a multi-vitamin ensures this. Two days really is a small sacrifice for attaining the body and quality of life you've always wanted, agreed?*

# Five "Free" Days Explained

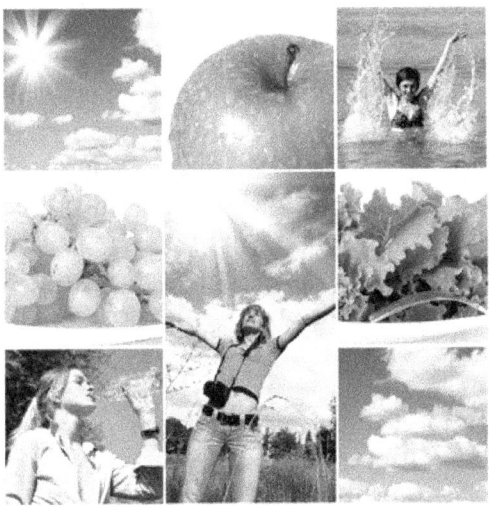

Keep in mind here if your goal is to lose weight, you really can't afford to go nuts on your five "unrestricted" days. Eating healthy is essential in any weight loss strategy. If you want to set yourself up for weight-loss success it's critical that you eat healthy with "Mediterranean Style" cuisine. This includes:
* Sticking to natural foods that aren't processed or packaged
* Fill up your tank with fresh fruits and vegetables
* Eating plenty of good carbs (complex carbohydrates) - whole grain breads, pastas, rice
* Also eat protein and fiber rich bean
* Include nuts and healthy oils (unsaturated, olive oil)
* Eating fish, skinless chicken, low-fat dairy
* Small amounts of lean cuts red meat

Specialty Note: Steer clear of or take it easy on pasta, red wine and pizza items! They're high is sugar, calories and fat for the most part.

How Much Do You Get To Eat?

The good news is that for five days you get to eat very well, around 1,800 calories worth. This is a HUGE step up from the 650 calories on your restricted days. This works to trigger your body physically and mentally to start burn more fat and calories than it would otherwise. By eating plenty of nutritious foods you are teaching your body it can trust you again. Something fad diets steal from you. And without trust you are going to battle your body to drop fat every inch of the way.

Eat well and healthy and your body is going to want to work with you to zap fat, energize you, deter disease and leave you with a perma-frown-turned-upside-down. Make sense?

You are also going to feel rewarded or special because you are able to eat more. Triggering your genuine appreciation for healthy food because you are regularly reminded of what it's like to have a little bit less than you want. So you aren't going extreme here, which is an inevitable disaster fact with most diets. It's like having half a glass of water for a couple days when you would have preferred a full cup. Bearable but not unbearable, leaving you elated with the five days you get your full glass.

Sample "Free Days"

DAY THREE
Breakfast
1 cup low-fat yogurt

1/2 cup fresh berries
1 slice whole grain toast with 1 tbsp all-natural peanut butter
Tea/water
Snack
Banana

Health Tip - By eating smaller meals throughout the day you are going to keep blood sugars level, energy constant, and encourage your body to burn more fat and calories on a routine basis. Regular healthy snacking is a good thing in moderation.

Lunch
1 boiled egg
2 cups spinach, 1 cup Romaine lettuce, 1 oz cheese, carrots, peppers, cucumbers, cherry tomatoes, 1/4 cup sunflower seeds, 1/4 cup raisins, 1 orange diced, drizzle olive oil based dressing
Flavored water
Snack
Cheese string
Dinner
1 4-6 oz grilled chicken breast
Whole grain roll
2 cups steamed mixed vegetables
Tea/Water
Snack
Veggie sticks
2 pieces fresh fruit

DAY FIVE
Breakfast
1 cup cooked oatmeal with 1/2 cup milk
1 apple sliced
1 cup low-fat milk
Coffee/tea/water

Snack
Handful nuts

Lunch
1 whole wheat tortilla with cucumber, tomato, lettuce, green peppers, red peppers, onions, 1 oz low-fat cheese, barbecue sauce or mustard to taste
3/4 cup low-fat cottage cheese or yogurt with 1/2 cup sliced peaches, mango or pineapple
Water/flavored water/tea

Snack
6-8 whole grain crackers with 1 tbsp all-natural peanut butter

Dinner
1 serving grilled salmon served on 2 cups spinach
1 cup cooked vegetables
3/4 cup whole grain rice
Water/Tea

Snack
2 x 2 inch cube cheese
1 apple, pear, or banana

Keep in mind that fresh vegetables and fruits should fill your plate first. Add to that a little bit of lean protein, including milk, cheese, yogurt, cottage cheese, skinless chicken, fish, or lean beef and some good carbohydrates, healthy whole grains, brown rice and pasta or beans. You should be eating healthy foods in moderation. This is a solid base from which to build and the more comfortable you get with this style of eating the more versatile it will be.

*My Thoughts . . .*

*This diet is strategically designed to actually teach you to appreciate and respect what it feels like to eat healthy and recognize moderation. Shifting from a small two day phase where you may not be eating the amount you'd like, to five days of getting lots ensures you appreciate the healthy foods you are eating and why you are eating them. It's not about externally triggered eating, emotions, hormones, habit or social pressures. You are learning to eat for your body and for energy and well-being, nothing else. Let me tell you something that feels absolutely wonderful.*

# The Mental "How To" Make the Two Day Diet Work

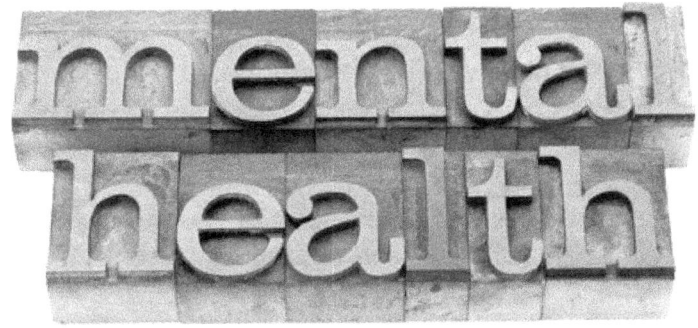

It doesn't matter what sort of new diet you are on. Dieting means change and as humans we are resistant to change. We are creatures of habit and find comfort in our routine, healthy or not. So in order to set yourself up for success and get off the "yo-yo dieting train," and onto the sustainable and effective weight loss two day diet to lose fat, fight off disease, and build you mentally and physically strong, you need to truly WANT it.

If you are just planning on going through the motions or maybe trying to lose fat for someone other than yourself, then don't both because it's not going to work. Change is hard and if you want to succeed in bettering your "self" for the long-term, you need to be completely on board with it.

Here are a few steps you need to take in order to get your mental on board with making your "Two Day Diet" a success for life.

* Know Why You Are Doing the Two Day Diet
It's time to come clean with exactly why you want to diet or simply change your lifestyle. Is it because you are seriously overweight? You're getting married in a few months and have a few pounds to lose? Or maybe you have developed some health issues that warrant you making some positive lifestyle changes a.s.a.p.? Make a list and reflect on it.

* Make Your Plan
Before starting the diet take a look at your lifestyle and schedule so you can set yourself up for success. Figure out which 2 days work best for your restrictive days. Many choose Monday and Tuesday to get started.
You can also plan your meals if you like to be organized. This means you don't have to think about what you'd like to eat when you're starving.

* Buy Your Weekly Food
It works well by making your weekly shopping list and buying all your food for the week in one shot. This will help you stick to the plan and get into your new routine.

* Prep Food
Set aside some time to prep food for the week if you can. Cut up all your veggies. You can also pre-cook any meat you are having if you like.

* Tell the World
The accountability factor is something you can never underestimate. If other people know you are using the "Two Day Diet," this is going to help you make your new

healthy habit stick. Most of us have no trouble disappointing ourselves, but it's a lot tougher to let other people down.

* Record It
I know this can be a bit of a pain in the rear. But people need to see progress and measure it to ensure effort equates to results. Keeping a consistent record of the changes you are making is going to inspire you to stick with it. You'll be able to look back and actually "see" that your positive lifestyle changes are getting you results. Losing fat, gaining strength mentally and physically and feeling fabulous for it.

* Plan Exercise
It's well known that regular exercise is going to help you build lean muscle and burn fat off faster. Muscle burns more calories that fat does and actually increases your resting metabolic rate, the rate in which you burn fat. Start with the basics and work your way up. 30 minutes 5-6 days a week of moderate cardiovascular exercise, like biking, walking, swimming, or an aerobics class is great. Incorporate 15 minutes of strength training or weights 2-3 times a week and you're off to a good start. Run this past your doctor first just to be safe and make sure you have a qualified fitness instructor set you up for success. The last thing you want to do is hurt yourself and end up sidelined.

* Set Up Rewards
You should be rewarded for your efforts and making positive changes in your eating with the "Two Day Diet." Now I don't mean you should hit the buffet after every ten pounds you drop. Talk about defeating the purpose here. But you should sit down and figure out what sort of reward you would like and put it into action. Maybe you want to buy a new pair of sexy jeans or a new workout

outfit after losing your first ten pounds? Perhaps you will set your reward on time frame instead, regardless of your progress? So every first Monday of the month you could go to the spa, get your hair done or maybe treat yourself to a show or something else you enjoy but never get to do very often.

The idea here is to make yourself feel special for making a commitment to positive health changes and sticking with it. Why? Just because you deserve it!

* Regular Check Ins
You head is a huge part of your success with the "Two Day Diet." It's important that you make the time to stop and reflect on your progress regularly. It doesn't have to take a whole lot of time but you do need to reaffirm your commitment to change and be okay in it. Sort of like re-minding yourself you're doing this for all the right reasons and it's very important that you renew this belief and keep on progressing forward one step at a time.

Pat yourself on the back and be proud of your accom-plishments no matter how "small" they are. If you lost five pounds of fat since your last "check-in," you should feel great about this. It may not be something other people notice but that's okay because it's important nonetheless.

*My Thoughts . . .*
*If you mentally prepare yourself for making a change in your eating you are one step closer to succeeding. In other words, you need to think and prepare yourself for the challenges that lay ahead. By taking the time to plan how you are going to execute your plan of action, goals and expectations, this will help you make the commit-ment and believe in yourself that you can open your mind to changes so that you can lose fat, gain energy, get*

*healthy and decrease your risk of developing serious disease.*

*Prevention is the key and the "Two Day Diet" sets you up to lose fat sensibly, which is linked directly to various diseases, including Breast Cancer, which has numerous studies that support this theory. Your mental happiness or mindset is going to make or break any health changes you attempt. Envision your "plan" with the "Two Day Diet," make sure you are open to making adjustments, and whatever you do DON'T give up if you are serious about getting leaner, healthier and happier for life!*

# Tips to Get Fit

Your body was made to be physically active every day of your life. Unfortunately time passed and we've created so many conveniences and techno-savvy devices that have eliminated the need to get off the couch and get active!

It's crazy how lazy our society has gotten and unfortunately this has caused our world to get fat and very unhealthy. By fitting regular physical activity into your life, something you enjoy and can commit to, you're going to gain trust from your body that will help you zap fat, gain energy, minimize pesky aches and pains, and deter disease from ruining your independent lifestyle, to start anyway.

Let's rewind the clock a touch a few hundred years ago, just after "cave-man" days. Every single thing in life required actually physical effort. There were no cell phones where a father could just ring up the local pizza shop and have dinner delivered without exerting any more energy than it took to dial the number. Oh, and he would have to get up and walk five steps to the door to actually get the pizza. Talk about LAZY!

Back in time if you were hungry you had to hop on your horse, if you were lucky, with your bow and arrow or spear and go track down dinner. If you were lucky you might come across a pack of gazelles and find one that is old, sick or wounded. Assuming you had lots of energy and perfect aim, you may get the kill.

But you're not done yet because now you had to drag your fresh dinner back five miles to camp and start the cleaning and cooking process. Actually I think the women usually got the honors here, but that doesn't mean the man was done. There were still trees that needed to be cut down and dragged back to camp for the fire, dishes that may need to be made and anything else you can think of that was required to eat. If there was time he might be able to slip a quick nap in by the berry patch but not likely.

Later that night the food would be ready to feast and by morning, your stomach would be growling again and the process would start all over again. Back then people were looking for breaks from strenuous physical activity. Not like today where we are looking to find time from our laziness to fit in some much needed exercise.
Here are a few pointers to help slip some regular exercise into your day:

* Motivation - If you are going to implement a successful exercise regimen into your life you are going to need to get motivated to do so. It's best if your motivation is inter-

nal. External motivators like a new boyfriend or family health scare will come and go and you need constant!

Working out with a friend will help to at least get you motivated to start. Remembering the first step is always the hardest. Hooking up your exercise with family outings is also a great method of motivation. Setting out specific days of the week to go biking or hiking is one step towards your health and wellness goals.

Maybe a pair of skinny jeans hanging in your closet from days past is motivation enough for you to turn off the snooze in the morning and get your butt out of bed to hit the gym and get your heart rate and energy levels up? You know you and it's critical you find your motivation and tap into it because the best is yet to come if you want it.

* Slow and Steady Wins the Race - It's true. If you want to be successful in fitting regular exercise into your life you are going to have to start slow and set yourself up for success. Recognize your tolerances and preferences and don't deny them. If you hate the thought of training in a gym setting, then don't! Try biking outside and doing weights at home. Or maybe you'd like to try an outdoor boot camp training session instead. Effective interval training progressing at your own pace by alternating intense cardio exercise, diverse weight training and strength training in a positive and motivational group setting is what's important here. Join a biking club or take aqua aerobics if you enjoy becoming one with the water. The bottom line is you need to do physical activities you enjoy or can honestly learn to enjoy. You're only kidding yourself if you are trying to make a permanent life change with an activity you detest. And yes, sex can qualify as an exercise, but we'll leave that one alone for now.

* Diversity

Diversity is the key in any long-term fitness regimen. Diversity means you aren't going to get bored, go through the motions or plateau, all of which are frustrating.

Boredom is something that triggers people to quit. If you walk on the treadmill every day at the exact same pace for the exact same amount of time, you're going to get bored. Your body is also going to memorize and predict your actions and start getting lazy by burning the minimum amount of energy required for your lazy walk. Top this off with hitting a plateau. You'll be putting in your daily efforts and seeing little or no results because your body and mind are in "Sleepville."

Change up your exercise routine and all your problems are solved. Even just changing the incline and/or pace in which you walk will kick your metabolism in the butt and tell it to burn more fat. Change also means your mind has to stay sharp and alert and this is going to starve off boredom. Make sense?

*My Thoughts . . .*

*You were born to exercise, that's a fact. I don't care whether you are 25 or 85, fit as a fiddle or a rather large piece of "flubber," you are only going to better you physical and mental with regular exercise. Start slow and do a little experimenting to see what works for you. Just because you don't like hiking with your buddies doesn't mean you should give up on exercise. All you need to do is keep trying things until you find physical exercise that you enjoy and get sweaty from.*

*It's mind over matter here and I promise you that if you stick with it and make it routine you will get results. Combined with the "Two Day Diet," you're going to. . .*

*\* zap fat*

*\* tone and strengthen muscles*

40

* increase energy
* increase mobility
* decrease aches and pains
* lower the risk of injury
* improve cognitive capacity
* improve relationships
* naturally increase your metabolic rate
* boost confidence and self-esteem
* make it spicier between the sheets
* lower the risk of disease and serious illness
* reduce anxiety and depression
* increase life expectancy

# Proven Strategies to Maintain

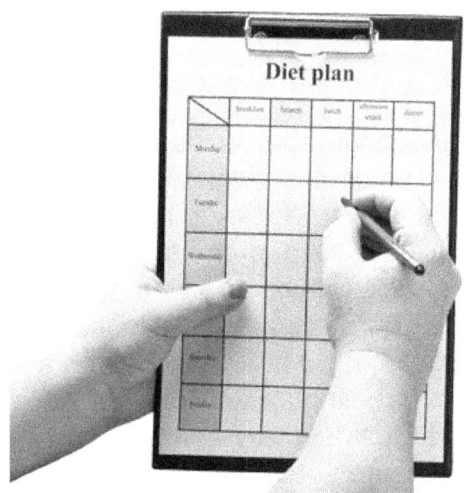

Losing weight and staying healthy isn't a walk in a park. It starts with change and change is something humans seem to naturally resist. Right or wrong that's just how the cookie crumbles. The "Two Day Diet" is a great way to drop fat and get healthy for the long run. If you want to do this you will. That's a fact. Here are a few strategies to help you stick with the program and maintain your weight loss and health benefits.

* ROUTINE
As creatures of habit we love routine and if you can stick with this diet long enough to make it a great new habit, you are setting yourself up for life-long success. Theoretically it takes at least 6 weeks of repeating a new habit consistently, in order to transform it into your new "nor-

43

mal," or a new healthy habit. In other words you've got to give yourself a chance to get used to your new eating style and allow your mind to adjust to the newness of it all. It will get more natural and comfortable in time and when this starts happening, when you start seeing results and you don't have to stop and think about what you should be eating, how much and when, that's when you've made progress.

* ACCOUTABILITY

Holding yourself accountable for our actions is important if you are making positive changes to your eating. There are many different ways people do this. Some use their weight and each week step on the scale and make certain they are on track. Maybe you want to use the clothing test. Are your "fat pants" still loose on you or are they starting to get snug. Maybe you'll keep a diary and go on how you are feeling as a whole.
The key here is to make sure you have something concrete that will measure your success, fast or slow doesn't matter as long as you are moving forward positively.

* FORGIVENESS

This one gets people into trouble. Life happens and sometimes we get thrown a curveball or two when we were expecting a fast ball down the middle. It's okay if you slip up here and there. You are human aren't you? What's important is not that you ate two hundred more calories than you should of, but that you recognize and admit this, and get yourself back on track right away. What happened in the past is done and finished and unless you've got a time-capsule you can't go back and change it. Yikes, that would cause a whole lot of problems
!
By absorbing your little steps back you are going to go stronger forward because you are excepting of your reali-

ty and understand the only way the "Two Day Diet" can fail you is if you quit on yourself. That isn't an option so all is good!

## * TROUBLE SHOOT

Recognizing things that might get in the way of your success before the fact is important. Maybe you have trouble saying no and dealing with peer pressure in social situations. So you might have to rethink heading out with the gang on Saturday nights because you know you're going to go extreme and end up feeling guilty in the morning. Now this doesn't mean removing yourself from your social life. But you do have to look out for yourself and recognize what's important to you. Where there's a will there's a way and you will figure it out.

Another example is maybe you are an emotional eater and know that if you're upset from work or you just got dumped, you're going to head to the junk food isle and sit at home filling your face for the night. Stop yourself and figure out a way to change this learned habit. If you are upset from work you could call a friend and go for a hike and talk about it instead of trying to eat the stress away. Do you see where I'm coming from? Be smart and look to prevent interference instead of dealing with it after the fact.

*My Thoughts . . .*
*You deserve to lose weight, gain energy and be healthy and happy. In order for the "Two Day Diet" to be successful long-term you need to make certain you commit to doing this. It's all about making small steps forward one at a time. Throw in a whole lot of patience and persistence and positive attitude and you are setting yourself up to maintain your progress.*
*Learn to look at the "big picture" instead of only the moment in time. It needs to make sense to you and you*

*need to feel and see that you are gaining value from this new way of eating. Don't sweat the little things and always keep your mind open to learning and implementing the new. Ask questions of a qualified expert when they arise and make certain you clear them up. Otherwise they will manifest into clutter and this will interfere with your progress and goals. You can do it!*

# Myths/Truths in the Diet World

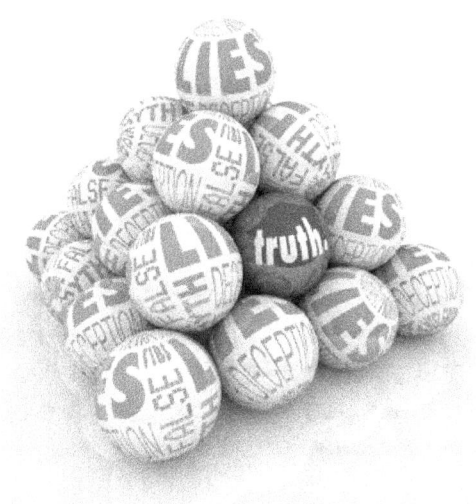

If I had a penny for every diet fib out there I'd have enough money for you and I to retire right now and then some! What's important here is not to focus on all the mistruths out there but rather to start nipping them in the bud and get the facts. Good or bad if you've got facts you can make better health decisions.

Myth One - Consuming caffeine is unhealthy.

Truth - Experts have discovered that caffeine is actually positive with regards to specific diseases. Gout and Parkinson's for example are positively affected by caffeine. Of course we are all familiar with the infamous "pick-me-up" or caffeine and truth be told, caffeine does NOT dehydrate you.

As with everything moderation is the key.

Myth Two - Drinking water helps get rid of fat.

Truth - Sorry to say there's no evidence that water triggers fat loss. But chin up because water does help you feel fuller and this will deter your system from eating as much. Just remember that feeling hungry and thirsty are two different things.

Myth Three - Protein is the most important type of nutrient for professional athletes.

Truth - Protein is a macronutrient that isn't manufactured by the body and it really can't be stored. This means you need to eat it regularly because your body needs it to function optimally. Protein is used to build lean muscle and of course that's something athletes are building and maintaining on a routine basis.

Bottom line is that athletes do need a little more protein than the average Joe. What's more important is when they have it. Before, sometimes during, depending on the length of training and intensity level, and always after during the recovery time is a must. So maybe a chicken breast with a whole grain wrap and cheese a few hours before training is a great mini-meal to fuel the body. After the workout or during the recovery time a light snack with protein and complex carbs is critical to rebuild energy stores and replenish lost nutrients from the exertive training session. A piece of whole grain toast with peanut butter and a dish of berries should do the trick.

Myth Four - All bread is created equal.

Truth - Sorry that's just not the case. Bread is a carbohydrate and there are 2 different types; complex and simple.

A simple carbohydrate is broken down into sugar quickly. Meaning it gives you a short burst of energy and then sends your energy levels straight down to the bottom of the barrel. White bread is a simple carb with very little nutritional value and only a minute amount of energy. Definitely the only exception to this is fruits, which are simple carbs, but the sugar is natural and they are loaded with essential vitamins and minerals that your body needs. Fruits are a form of simple carbohydrates that do your body good.

Complex carbohydrates are your best choice. Multigrain breads are a form or complex carbohydrates and are full of essential nutrients, lots of healthy fiber and this extends the duration of energy provided by eating them. Choosing to eat these carbs are going to help level your blood sugars and keep your moods in check, you'll feel fuller longer and you are energizing your system to train longer and harder. Examples are brown breads, pasta and rice, sweet potato and various other vegetables.

Myth Five - Yo-yo dieting is going to screw up your chances of losing weight long-term.

Truth - Just because you are human like everyone else on the planet and have tried at least a few different fad diets, doesn't mean you are stuck in on the roller coaster of weight loss and gain forever.

Anyone can hop of this roller coaster whenever they decide to commit to making new healthy eating habits and stick with them. The "Two Day Diet" will help reprogram your mind and body to work together in helping you zap fat, deter disease, and get healthy for life. It's a process you need to take one step at a time and stick with it. This is the only way you are going to get the body you want and mind to match and enjoy your hard work for the rest of your days. You are worth it!

Myth Six - In order to avoid developing cardiovascular disease you should use margarine instead of butter.

Truth - Fact is that studies show people consuming margarine are twice as likely to develop cardiovascular disease. The Trans fats in many margarines are worse for your health than "bad" saturated fats. The one exception to this rule, in moderation of course, is coconut oil. It's considered a saturated fat but has so many health benefits the pros definitely outweigh the cons.

FOODS TO AVOID IN GENERAL AS THEY CAN BE TOXIC FOR YOUR BODY, PARTICULARLY IN LARGE AMOUNTS

* Processed foods like cakes, pastries, crackers, soda, packaged dinners etc.
* White flour and products
* Hydrogenated fats and oils
* Trans fat
* Fried food
* Salad Dressing and high fat condiments like mayonnaise
* Lunch meats and other processed meats including hotdogs
* Cooking sprays
* Manufactured food additives, particularly MSG
* Anything that has an unnatural shelf life - like banana bread that's good for a month
* Creamy sauces and soups, stick with clear soups and tomato sauce

* Fatty meats
* Sugary juices and drinks

*My Thoughts . . .*

*As mentioned previous there are all sorts of rumors floating around about what you should and shouldn't eat. When you stop and think about it the "indecision" in the air is enough to make your head spin. Hopefully this has cleared up at least a few of the rumors you may have heard so that you can make smarter decisions when it comes to your eating and great health. It's a start anyway.*

# Final Thoughts

Your health matters . . . You matter. It's important you do everything you can to keep your body healthy, strong and disease-free, so that you live your life to the fullest every day. Unfortunately, many of us take our good health for granted and suddenly it gets taken from us. The "Two Day Diet" gives you the knowledge, scientific validation, and the practical logic to change your eating habits for the better and stick with it.

By learning to appreciate what you are eating and teaching yourself how great it feels to eat nutritiously, you are setting into motion a very important health change. It's one that will set you up for long-term weight loss success.

With the combination of restricting your eating while still getting the essential vitamins and minerals your body requires, and rewarding it with five days of "free' healthy eating, you are re-programming your learned eating habits for the better. If you really want to change for the better, lose weight, gain strength and increase your resistance to serious disease, in particular cancer. Then you have to get your "mental" ready to accept and stick with reasonable change. This isn't about jumping off the bridge and hoping for the best, like most other diets out there. The "Two Day Diet" is a scientific opportunity to give your body what it needs to trust you, help you zap fat and build up resistance to disease, all while feeling energized and optimistic.

You need to get uncomfortable to get comfortable and understand there is no "perfect" diet out there for anyone.

You need to gather information and use the aspects of the "Two Day Diet" that work for you. The concept is genius, but that doesn't really matter. It only matters if you understand it and more importantly apply it. Not just for a week or two but for life.

This is about committing to change. Opening your mind to a different avenue to reach your health and wellness goals. What do you say? It's worth giving a shot don't you agree?

We have the choice to look for the positive or the negative in life. You can choose to lift someone up or to stomp on them. Writing is my passion and I work hard at it, with the goal of helping make people better. If you gain a new piece of knowledge, read something that makes you think, or perhaps even smile a few times, then I am happy and content!

Life's just too short not to tune into optimism. If your glass is half full, then I invite you to read my writing, and if you have a minute to spare when you're through, **I would appreciate your review.** This will help me better myself and my writing. I thank you in advance and appreciate you.